Sensei Self Development

Mental Health Chronicles Series

An Introduction To Mindfulness

Sensei Paul David

Copyright Page

Sensei Self Development -
An Introduction To Mindfulness,
by Sensei Paul David

Copyright © 2023

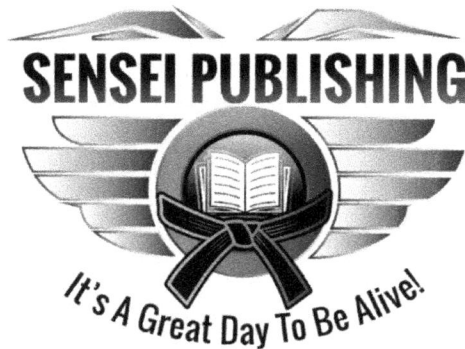

SENSEI PUBLISHING

It's A Great Day To Be Alive!

www.senseipublishing.com

@senseipublishing
#senseipublishing

Get/Share Your FREE SSD Mental Health Chronicles at
www.senseiselfdevelopment.care

or

CLICK HERE

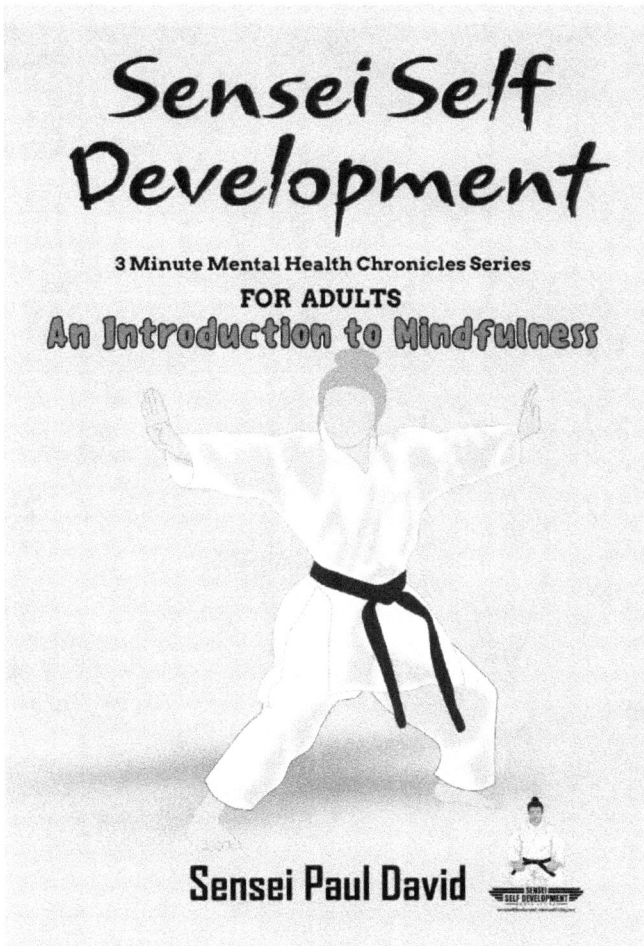

Check Out The SSD Chronicles Series CLICK HERE

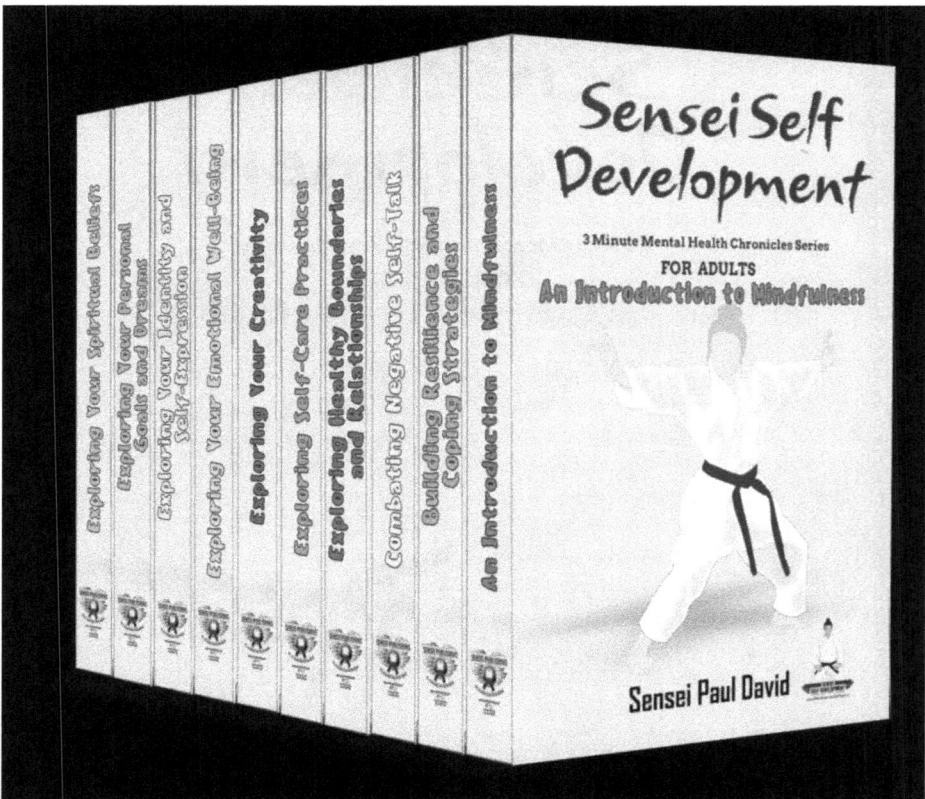

Dedication

To those who courageously take action towards self-improvement - you are helping to evolve the world for generations to come.

- It's a great day to be alive!

If Found Please Contact:

_____

Reward If Found:

_____

MY
COMMITMENT

I, _____

commit to writing This Sensei Self Development Journal for at least 10 days in a row, starting: _____

Writing this journal is valuable to me because:

_____

_____

_____

_____

_____

_____

If I finish a minimum of 10 consecutive days of writing in this journal, I will reward myself by:

_____

_____

_____

_____

_____

_____

If I don't finish 10 days of writing this journal, I will promise to:

_____

_____

_____

_____

_____

_____

I will do the following things to ensure that I write in my Sensei Self Development Journal every day:

_____

_____

_____

_____

_____

_____

Get/Share Your FREE All-Ages Mental Health eBook Now at

www.senseiselfdevelopment.com

Or CLICK HERE

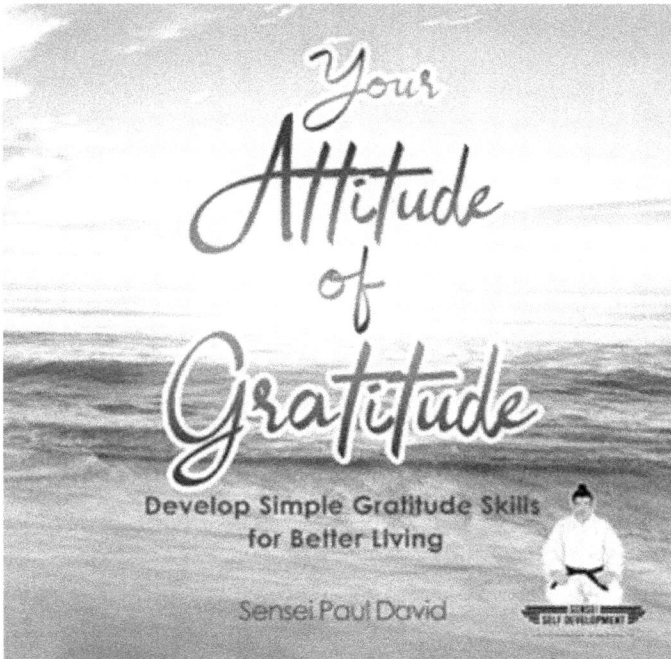

senseiselfdevelopment.com

Check Out Another Book In The
SSD BOOK SERIES:

senseipublishing.com/SSD_SERIES

CLICK HERE

SENSEI
SELF DEVELOPMENT
B O O K S   S E R I E S

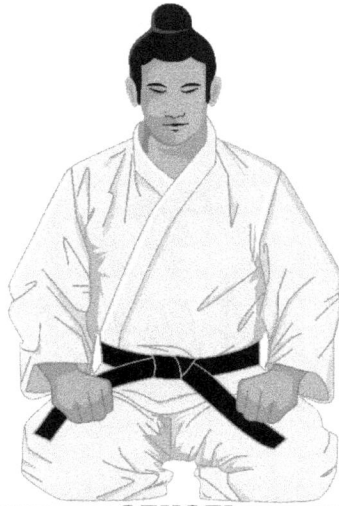

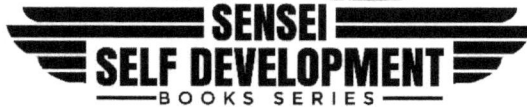

senseiselfdevelopment.senseipublishing.com

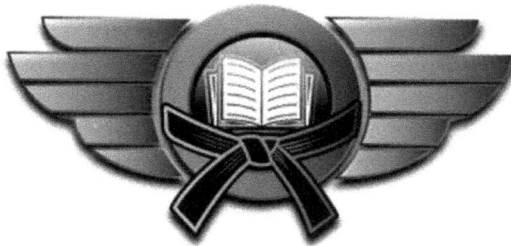

Join Our Publishing Journey!

If you would like to receive FUTURE FREE BOOKS and get to know us better, please click www.senseipublishing.com and join our newsletter by entering your email address in the pop-up box.

Follow Our Blog: senseipauldavid.ca

Follow/Like/Subscribe: Facebook, Instagram, YouTube: @senseipublishing

Scan the QR Code with your phone or tablet

to follow us on social media: Like / Subscribe / Follow

A Message From The Author:
Sensei Paul David

Dear Reader,

Welcome to the world of mental health journaling – a sacred space for self-reflection, growth, and healing. Within these pages, you hold the power to uplift your spirit, invigorate your mind, and nourish your goals.

In a world that often moves at blink-and-you'll-miss-it speed, it's crucial to make time for self-care and self-discovery.

Anxiety, stress, and emotional turbulence may have clouded your mind, making it difficult to find clarity and peace within. But fear not! Together, we will navigate the labyrinth of emotions, and experiences, helping to simplify the path to mental well-being.

This journal is not merely a bunch of blank pages awaiting your words. It is your compassionate companion, offering solace and understanding during your unique journey. Here, you are free to unburden yourself, celebrate small and large victories, and confront the challenges that may still linger.

Within the sheltered realm of these pages, there is no judgment, no expectation, and no pressure. Your unique experience and perspective hold immeasurable worth, and your voice deserves to be heard. Whether you choose to fill the lines with eloquence or simply scribble fragments of your thoughts, please remember each entry is a valuable contribution to your growth.

In this sacred space, you are challenged to take off the mask we so often wear in the outside world. It is here that you can be raw, vulnerable, and authentic – allowing your true self to be seen and embraced without reservation. By giving yourself permission to explore the depths of your emotions and confront the shadows that may lurk within, you will discover profound insights and find the healing you seek over time.

As you embark on this journaling journey, I encourage you to embrace the process itself rather than fixate solely on the outcome. Remember, it is not about reaching a certain destination or ticking off boxes on a list of accomplishments. Rather, it is about cultivating self-awareness, fostering self-compassion, and nurturing a sense of curiosity about the intricate workings of your intelligently beautiful mind.

In the quiet moments of reflection, let your pen become a bridge between your inner world and the possibilities that lie ahead. Create a sanctuary for your thoughts, fears, triumphs, and dreams. As you pour your heart onto these pages, allow your words to be a living testament to courage, resilience, and an unwavering commitment to your own well-being.

I am honored to be a part of your journey, and I believe in your ability to navigate the twists and turns with grace and resilience. Remember, you are not alone in this – countless others have walked similar paths, faced similar challenges, and emerged stronger and wiser on the other side. You have the power to reclaim all of your untapped joy, cultivate a positive mindset that serves you, and foster a deep sense of self-love and peaceful confident. – And it will take a worth effort and time.

So, open the first page of this journal with hope, curiosity, and an open heart and open mind. Embrace the transformative power of self-reflection, and allow it to guide you towards a life of greater fulfilment and peace. Each journaling session is an opportunity to not only connect with yourself but also to rekindle the light within that sometimes flickers but never extinguishes.

Remember, the pages you are about to fill are not just a record of your journey but also a testament to your strength, resilience, and indomitable spirit. Cherish this space, invest in yourself, and let your words be an ode to the magnificent journey of becoming whole.

With great respect for your decision to evolve,

Paul

MY CONVICTION

Please circle your answers below

I am DECIDING to be patient with myself and this PROCESS each time I journal toward my improved state of mental well-being

YES   NO

"The present moment is filled with joy and happiness. If you are attentive, you will see it."

Thich Nhat Hanh

Introduction

Mindfulness means being awake. It means knowing what you are doing – Jon Kabat-Zinn

Imagine walking through a bustling, vibrant jungle. Your senses are overwhelmed by the cacophony of sounds and the flurry of movement. In this jungle lives a little monkey, let's name her Mia. She's agile, energetic, and constantly on the move, her eyes darting from one shiny object to another, her hands grabbing at every fruit and leaf within reach. Mia is much like your mind, always active, always grasping after thoughts, worries, and desires.

Now, as you wander deeper into the jungle, you notice how Mia jumps frantically from branch to branch, never resting, never still. You see her chasing after butterflies, only to lose interest the moment she catches them. This endless pursuit leaves her exhausted, yet she can't seem to stop. Isn't this familiar? Like Mia, your mind often races from one thought to another, seeking happiness in a relentless stream of desires and fears, finding little peace.

As the sun sets, you stumble upon a hidden glade, a place of remarkable stillness and calm. In the center, there's a crystal-clear pond, its surface smooth as glass. Curiously, Mia follows you there and, for the first time, you see her sit quietly, mesmerized by the still water. She seems to forget her endless chase, her body relaxes, and a sense of peace envelops her.

This glade, this moment of tranquillity, is the essence of mindfulness. It's a state where the mind, like Mia, stops chasing every fleeting thought and desire. It rests in the present, acknowledging and observing, but not grasping. In this stillness, there's no suffering from relentless pursuit, no exhaustion from the chase. There's just peace, clarity, and an understanding of the nature of your thoughts.

As you leave the jungle with Mia at your side, calmer and more composed, you realize that this serene glade isn't a physical place. It's a state of being, accessible to you anytime, anywhere.

Mindfulness is a mental practice that involves focusing your awareness on the present moment while calmly acknowledging and accepting your feelings, thoughts, and bodily sensations.

Mindfulness is a way of being that invites us to pause and notice the world around us, and more importantly, the world within us. Picture yourself sitting quietly, perhaps in a favorite chair or under a tree, letting go of the rush of thoughts about yesterday or tomorrow. Instead, you focus on the here and now: the rhythm of your breath, the sensations in your body, the sounds of life happening around you.

Mindfulness isn't about emptying your mind or achieving some mystical state; it's more about welcoming everything just as it is. Think of it as sitting by a river, watching your thoughts and feelings float by like leaves on the water. You don't need to chase them or hold onto them; you simply acknowledge their presence and let them drift away.

In daily life, mindfulness can be as simple as truly tasting your food, feeling the sun on your skin, or listening to a friend without planning what to say next. It's about being fully present in the small moments, which can lead to a greater sense of peace and connection.

And just like any skill, mindfulness grows with practice. Each time we choose to be present, we strengthen our ability to engage with the world in a more grounded, calm, and compassionate way. It's a journey of discovering the richness of the ordinary, and the extraordinary peace that comes from simply being.

A Brief History of Mindfulness

The roots of mindfulness are often traced back to ancient Buddhist teachings, particularly those of Siddhartha Gautama, the Buddha, who lived around the 5th century BCE. In Buddhism, mindfulness, known as 'sati' in Pali, is a key element in the practice of meditation and is integral to the Noble Eightfold Path, a guide to ethical and mindful living. The essence of mindfulness in Buddhism is to maintain a moment-by-moment awareness of our thoughts, feelings, bodily sensations, and the surrounding environment with a gentle, nurturing lens.

However, the concept of mindfulness is not exclusive to Buddhism. Similar practices can be found in other spiritual traditions, including Hinduism, Taoism, and various Christian contemplative practices. For instance, in Hinduism, mindfulness is a component of yoga, focusing on self-awareness and the connection between mind, body, and spirit.

The journey of mindfulness into Western consciousness began more prominently in the 20th century. One pivotal figure in this journey was Jon Kabat-Zinn, an American professor emeritus of medicine. In the 1970s, he founded the Mindfulness-Based Stress Reduction (MBSR) program at the University of Massachusetts Medical School. Kabat-Zinn's work was revolutionary in that it stripped mindfulness of religious and cultural trappings, presenting it in a secular, scientific context. His program demonstrated that mindfulness meditation could be an effective tool in managing stress, chronic pain, and a variety of other health issues.

This secular adaptation of mindfulness sparked a growing interest in the scientific community. Researchers began to explore its effects on the brain and body, leading to a surge in studies and publications on the topic. Neuroscientific research, for instance, has shown that mindfulness meditation can lead to changes in brain regions related to attention, emotion regulation, and self-awareness.

In the 21st century, mindfulness has permeated various aspects of modern life. It's found in schools, where it's used to help students focus and manage stress; in workplaces, to improve employee well-being and productivity; and even in the military, to enhance resilience and mental readiness. Mindfulness practices have diversified, including mindfulness-based cognitive therapy (MBCT), mindful eating, and various forms of mindfulness meditation.

The proliferation of digital technology has also played a role in spreading mindfulness. Apps and online programs have made mindfulness exercises more accessible to a broader audience, allowing individuals to practice in their own space and time.

Today, mindfulness stands as a testament to the human quest for peace, understanding, and connection. It bridges ancient wisdom and contemporary science, offering a path to navigate the complexities of modern life with greater calm and clarity. This journey, from ancient monasteries to modern smartphones, reflects our enduring desire to cultivate a deeper sense of awareness and harmony within ourselves and with the world around us.

Benefits of Mindfulness

1. Stress Reduction: Research has consistently shown that mindfulness significantly reduces stress. A 2010 study synthesized a decade of findings, confirming its efficacy in relieving

stress and anxiety, regardless of pre-existing conditions.

2. Enhanced Working Memory and Focus: A study from the University of California, Santa Barbara, revealed that mindfulness boosts focus and the ability to use new information. Notably, participants reported less mind wandering after just two weeks of mindfulness practice.

3. Physical Health Benefits: Over the past decade, research has linked mindfulness to improved digestion, a stronger immune system, lower blood pressure, faster healing, and decreased inflammation, underlining that mindfulness benefits the body as well as the mind.

4. Improved Sleep: Harvard Health reports that mindfulness aids in falling and staying asleep. Meditation practice can enhance sleep quality, irrespective of the time of day it's practiced.

5. Creative Problem Solving: A 1982 study highlighted that meditation

fosters creativity in problem-solving. Mindfulness helps in viewing challenges from new perspectives, thereby enhancing effectiveness in personal and professional problem-solving.

6. Reduction in Feelings of Loneliness: A University of California, Los Angeles, study found that eight weeks of mindfulness practice led to decreased feelings of loneliness. This effect was observed in both solitary individuals and those in social settings, suggesting that mindfulness fosters a deeper sense of connection.

7. Boosted Self-Esteem: Mindfulness practice has been shown to improve self-esteem across various cultures. It enhances body image, self-worth, and overall satisfaction with oneself.

8. Mood Regulation: While not a substitute for clinical treatment, mindfulness is effective in stabilizing mood disorders. It's been beneficial for individuals experiencing depression,

anxiety, or mood swings, both with and without diagnosed mood disorders.

Mindfulness in Daily Life

Incorporating mindfulness into daily life is like inviting a gentle, calming presence into every moment. It's about embracing the world with a sense of openness and attentiveness, whether you're engaged in routine tasks or facing new challenges.

Imagine starting your day with a few minutes of quiet mindfulness. As you wake, you take a moment to simply be aware of your breath, feeling its natural rhythm, noticing the rise and fall of your chest. This simple act sets a tone of calm and presence for your day.

As you go about your morning routine, mindfulness transforms ordinary activities into opportunities for awareness. While brushing your teeth or taking a shower, you focus on the sensations - the taste of the toothpaste, the sound of the water, the feeling of the brush or water against your skin. This practice of being fully present turns mundane tasks into moments of calm and connection.

Mindful eating is another beautiful practice. It involves eating slowly and without distraction, savoring each bite, and being fully present with the experience of eating. This not only enhances the enjoyment of your meal but also promotes better digestion and a deeper appreciation for the food.

Throughout the day, mindfulness can be a refuge. In moments of stress or busyness, pausing to take a few deep, conscious breaths can be profoundly centering. It's a way of grounding yourself, creating a small island of tranquility in the midst of a hectic day.

Mindfulness also enriches interactions with others. When you're fully present in a conversation, truly listening and engaging, it deepens your connection with others. It's about giving the gift of your attention, one of the most precious things you can offer.

As the day winds down, mindfulness can help in transitioning to rest. Reflecting on the day with gratitude, acknowledging both the highs and lows with a non-judgmental attitude, and then letting go, prepares you for a restful night.

Incorporating mindfulness into daily life doesn't require extra time or special circumstances. It's about the quality of attention you bring to each moment. It's a practice of returning, again and again, to the here and now, finding depth and richness in the simplicity of everyday life. This gentle, serene approach to living can transform your experience of the world, opening the door to a deeper sense of peace and connectedness.

Mindfulness Vs Mindful Meditation

Mindful meditation is a practice within the broader concept of mindfulness. It's a dedicated time for cultivating a deep and intentional awareness of the present moment. During mindful meditation, you typically find a quiet space to sit or lie down comfortably, and then focus your attention on something specific, often your breath, a word, or a sensation in your body.

As you engage in this practice, your mind will naturally wander. Thoughts, feelings, and sensations will arise. In mindful meditation, you observe these mental events with a gentle, non-judgmental attitude. Instead of getting caught up in your thoughts, you acknowledge them and then gently redirect your attention back to your chosen point of focus, like your breath.

This practice of returning your attention to the present moment is at the heart of mindful meditation. It's not about achieving a state of total emptiness or constant tranquility in your mind, but rather about practicing the skill of paying attention, of being aware of your experience without getting lost in it.

By regularly engaging in mindful meditation, you cultivate a heightened sense of awareness and presence. This practice strengthens your ability to be mindful in everyday life, enhancing your capacity to engage with the world in a more conscious, calm, and centered way. Mindful meditation, therefore, is a key component of mindfulness, offering a structured approach to developing the skills of attention and presence that are central to living mindfully.

The Science of Mindfulness

Mindfulness and Happiness

Study 1: Mindfulness Meditation and Psychological Well-being (2011)

In 2011, researchers Keng, Smoski, and others delved into how mindfulness meditation affects our psychological well-being. Their comprehensive review brought to light these key findings:

- Enhanced Well-being: They discovered that mindfulness meditation significantly boosts well-being. It plays a crucial role in increasing happiness, reducing anxiety, and lessening symptoms of depression.

- Improved Emotional Regulation: Importantly, mindfulness aids in better emotional regulation. This is vital for maintaining a positive mood and overall happiness.

Study 2: Mindfulness-Based Stress Reduction and Happiness (2010)

Nyklíček and Kuijpers in 2010 explored the effects of Mindfulness-Based Stress Reduction (MBSR) on happiness. Their findings were enlightening:

- Increased Happiness: Participants experienced a substantial increase in happiness and positive affect after the 8-week MBSR program.

- Reduction in Negative Affect: The program also led to a decrease in negative emotions and stress, enhancing overall happiness and well-being.

Mindfulness and Anxiety

In 2013, Zeidan and his team examined how mindfulness meditation could alleviate anxiety, especially in those new to meditation. Their findings were encouraging:

- Reduction in Anxiety Levels: Even brief mindfulness meditation training significantly reduced reported anxiety levels.

- Brain Changes: Brain imaging revealed changes in brain areas linked to anxiety control. These changes corresponded with the reduction in anxiety, suggesting that short-term mindfulness practice can alter brain function in ways that reduce anxiety.

Mindfulness Meditation and Sleep Quality (2018)

Dr. Sarah Thompson's 2018 study focused on how mindfulness meditation affects sleep quality. The results were quite positive:

- Enhanced Sleep Quality: Participants, many of whom were experiencing sleep disturbances, reported improved sleep quality.

- Reduction in Sleep-Related Anxiety: The meditation also helped reduce sleep-related anxiety, contributing to better overall sleep quality.

Mindfulness Meditation and Physical Health

Study 1: In 2003, a groundbreaking study by Davidson and Kabat-Zinn revealed that mindfulness meditation could enhance the immune system. Key findings included:

- Enhanced Immune Function: Those practicing mindfulness showed a significant increase in immune response compared to the control group.

- Positive Emotional Changes: The meditation group also reported increased levels of positive emotions.

Study 2: Mindfulness-Based Stress Reduction and Chronic Pain (1985)

One of the earliest studies, conducted by Kabat-Zinn and colleagues in 1985, focused on chronic pain. Key findings:

- Reduction in Pain Symptoms: Most participants reported significant reductions in pain and improved coping abilities.

- Enhanced Quality of Life: Alongside pain reduction, there were improvements in mood and psychological well-being.

Mindfulness and Productivity

Study 1: Mindfulness Training and Workplace Productivity (2012)

This study explored the impact of mindfulness on workplace productivity. The key findings included:

- Increased Focus and Concentration: Participants reported improved concentration and focus.

- Reduced Stress and Improved Emotional Regulation: Mindfulness training helped reduce stress levels and enhance emotional regulation, leading to better workplace performance.

Study 2: Mindfulness Meditation and Executive Functioning (2016)

In 2016, Mrazek and colleagues investigated how mindfulness meditation affects cognitive functions. Their findings showed:

- Improved Executive Functioning: Short-term mindfulness training significantly improved aspects of executive functioning, including working memory and attentional control.

- Enhanced Task Performance: Participants demonstrated improved performance on tasks requiring executive functions.

EIGHT ASPECTS OF MINDFULNESS PRACTICE

You're here because you've decided to explore mindfulness, and that's a significant step worth celebrating. Give yourself a moment to appreciate your choice. As you begin your journey into mindfulness practice, let's examine the nine aspects you'll be cultivating:

1. **Being Fully Present:** This fundamental aspect of mindfulness involves staying in the present moment. It might take practice to keep bringing your mind back, but with time, being present becomes more natural.

2. **Seeing Clearly:** Mindfulness allows you to recognize your experiences for what they are. When you feel pain or anxiety, you learn to identify it as such, fostering clarity in the present moment.

3. **Letting Go of Judgment:** You might notice your mind labeling experiences as good or bad. In mindfulness, you learn to release these judgments and accept each moment as it is, including any feelings of preference or aversion.

4. **Being Equanimous:** This is about maintaining balance, especially in challenging situations. Mindfulness helps you approach experiences, whether easy

or difficult, with consistent energy and effort, building resilience.

5. **Allowing Everything to Belong:** As taught by Ajahn Sumedho, "Everything belongs." In mindfulness, you don't exclude any thoughts, emotions, or experiences. You make space for all, including the uncomfortable ones.

6. **Being Patient:** People often come to mindfulness with specific goals, like reducing anxiety or managing stress. It's important to be patient and trust in the process, your teacher, and yourself, allowing growth to happen naturally.

7. **Making a Friend:** Mindfulness involves kindness, especially towards yourself. Reacting with gentleness to your experiences is key, treating your mind as a friend rather than a foe.

8. **Respecting Yourself:** You don't have to be perfect to practice mindfulness. Start where you are and respect your own journey. This is about personal growth, not competition or achieving perfection. Struggles are part of the process and

don't mean there's something wrong with you or your mind.

Each of these aspects is integral to developing a mindful approach to life, helping you grow in awareness and understanding.

Starting a Mindfulness Practice

When I first got into mindfulness, it was kind of tough. I remember feeling like it was just another thing to squeeze into my day. But as I stuck with it, it sort of grew on me. I started looking forward to those quiet moments. The more I did it, the more it felt less like a chore and more like a cool part of my day. It's kind of amazing how something so simple can start making a difference in how you feel and see things.

Finding Time for It

Honestly, at first, it seemed impossible to find time for meditation. But it's really about just making it a priority. I began with just 5 minutes a day. Setting a specific time helped a lot, like a reminder on my phone or doing it first thing in the morning.

Your Own Space

Finding a good spot to meditate can be tricky. But really, you can do it anywhere. I used to think I needed a perfect quiet room or something, but I learned to let that go. Sometimes, I'd just find a calm spot in my house or even sit in my car for a bit before going into work.

Why Are You Doing It?

Setting an intention is pretty important. Like, why did you want to start practicing mindfulness in the first place? Keeping that in mind helps, especially when you're not really feeling like doing it.

Stick With It

Staying consistent makes a huge difference. It's like working out; you don't see the changes right away, but over time, it adds up. I tried to do something mindful every day, even if it was just for a few minutes.

Find a Buddy

Doing it with a friend or family member can be a big help. It's kind of like having a gym buddy. It keeps you on track, and it's nice to have someone to talk to about what you're experiencing.

Writing It Down

I started keeping a journal about my mindfulness stuff. After each session, I'd write a bit about how it went, what I noticed, or how I felt. Looking back at those notes now is pretty cool. It's like seeing a map of how far I've come.

How Do I Know It's Working?

When you first start mindfulness practice, it might not feel like much is happening. It's incredibly challenging to just sit still and observe the whirlwind of thoughts in your mind, particularly in the beginning. But remember, like any new habit, mindfulness takes time to show its effects. It's called a practice for a reason - it's not about reaching a finish line or completing a checklist. Think of mindfulness as a lifelong companion, not a quick fix.

As you continue with your practice, you'll start to notice moments of mindfulness sprinkling into your daily life. These moments are subtle yet powerful indicators that it's working. You might also find yourself craving immediate results or a magical 'cure' for your worries. When these thoughts arise, try to approach them with curiosity rather than impatience. This is part of the process - learning to let go and trust the journey you're on.

In the early stages of your mindfulness practice, it's all about laying the groundwork for a deeper understanding of your mind. So, if you're wondering whether it's working, pay attention to these small changes and shifts in your perspective. They are the seeds of a more mindful, aware, and peaceful existence that you're cultivating, one breath at a time.

Before We Get Started…

Remember, mindfulness journaling is a personal practice, and these questions are meant to guide and inspire you. Feel free to adapt and modify them to suit your needs and preferences. Explore, reflect, and embrace the opportunity to deepen your self-awareness and cultivate a sense of inner peace.

Date ___ / ___ / ___: S M T W Th F S

I feel:
(please circle)

because because because because because

_____ _____ _____ _____ _____
_____ _____ _____ _____ _____

Today I Am Grateful For

1. _____
2. _____
3. _____

What could help transform today into a remarkable day?

Reflective Writing
What am I feeling in this moment?

_____

_____

_____

_____

_____

_____

_____

_____

What is mindfulness?

a. A type of meditation
b. A way of being aware in the present moment
c. A form of mental exercise
d. A type of yoga

All Are Correct - Choose The Response You Feel Is Most Important To Remember

Date ___ / ___ / ___ : S   M   T   W   Th   F   S

I feel:
(please circle)

because _____   because _____   because _____   because _____   because _____

Today I Am Grateful For

1. _____
2. _____
3. _____

What could help transform today into a remarkable day?

Reflective Writing

What peaceful imagery can I think of to help relax my mind?

_____

_____

_____

_____

_____

_____

_____

_____

What is the purpose of practicing mindfulness?

a. To reduce stress and anxiety
b. To increase focus and concentration
c. To become more organized
d. To improve physical health

All Are Correct - Choose The Response You Feel Is Most Important To Remember

Date ___ / ___ / ___ : S M T W Th F S

I feel:
(please circle)

because _____ because _____ because _____ because _____ because _____

Today I Am Grateful For

1. _____
2. _____
3. _____

What could help transform today into a remarkable day?

Reflective Writing

What is something I can do to show myself kindness today?

_____

_____

_____

_____

_____

_____

_____

How can mindfulness be practiced?

a.   Through mindful breathing exercises
b.   Through mindful eating
c.   Through mindful walking
d.   All of the above

All Are Correct - Choose The Response You Feel Is Most Important To Remember

Date ___ / ___ / ___: S   M   T   W   Th   F   S

I feel:
(please circle)

because   because   because   because   because

_____ _____ _____ _____ _____

_____ _____ _____ _____ _____

Today I Am Grateful For

1. _____
2. _____
3. _____

What could help transform today into a remarkable day?

Reflective Writing

How can I bring more mindfulness into my daily routine?

_____

_____

_____

_____

_____

_____

_____

34

What type of thoughts can be experienced during mindfulness meditation?

a. Positive thoughts
b. Negative thoughts
c. Neutral thoughts
d. All of the above

All Are Correct - Choose The Response You Feel Is Most Important To Remember

Date ___ / ___ / ___ : S   M   T   W   Th   F   S

I feel:
(please circle)

because _____   because _____   because _____   because _____   because _____

Today I Am Grateful For

1. _____
2. _____
3. _____

What could help transform today into a remarkable day?

Reflective Writing

What is a negative thought or belief I have been holding onto? How can I challenge or reframe it?

_____

_____

_____

_____

_____

_____

_____

_____

What are the benefits of mindfulness?

a. Reduced stress and anxiety
b. Improved mental clarity and focus
c. Increased emotional awareness
d. All of the above

All Are Correct - Choose The Response You Feel Is Most Important
To Remember

Date ___ / ___ / ___ : S M T W Th F S

I feel:
(please circle)

because because because because because
_____ _____ _____ _____ _____
_____ _____ _____ _____ _____

Today I Am Grateful For

1. _____
2. _____
3. _____

What could help transform today into a remarkable day?

Reflective Writing

What is something I am struggling with or finding challenging in my life right now?

_____

_____

_____

_____

_____

_____

_____

_____

What type of environment is best for mindfulness practice?

a. Quiet and peaceful
b. Busy and noisy
c. Relaxing and comfortable
d. All of the above

All Are Correct - Choose The Response You Feel Is Most Important
To Remember

Date ___ / ___ / ___ : S   M   T   W   Th   F   S

I feel:
(please circle)

because _____   because _____   because _____   because _____   because _____

Today I Am Grateful For

1. _____
2. _____
3. _____

What could help transform today into a remarkable day?

Reflective Writing

How can I practice self-compassion and self-forgiveness today?

_____

_____

_____

_____

_____

_____

_____

_____

How often should mindfulness be practiced?

a. Once a day
b. Twice a day
c. Three times a day
d. As often as possible

All Are Correct - Choose The Response You Feel Is Most Important To Remember

Date ___ / ___ / ___ : S   M   T   W   Th   F   S

I feel:
(please circle)

because   because   because   because   because

_____   _____   _____   _____   _____

_____   _____   _____   _____   _____

Today I Am Grateful For

1. _____
2. _____
3. _____

What could help transform today into a remarkable day?

Reflective Writing

What is a recent situation that triggered strong emotions in me? How can I reflect on it and grow from it?

_____

_____

_____

_____

_____

_____

_____

What is the best way to begin a mindfulness practice?

a. Taking a few deep breaths
b. Listening to calming music
c. Setting a goal for the practice
d. All of the above

All Are Correct - Choose The Response You Feel Is Most Important To Remember

Date ___ / ___ / ___ : S   M   T   W   Th   F   S

I feel:
(please circle)

because   because   because   because   because
_____   _____   _____   _____   _____
_____   _____   _____   _____   _____

Today I Am Grateful For

1. _____
2. _____
3. _____

What could help transform today into a remarkable day?

Reflective Writing

What are some self-care activities I can engage in
to nurture my mind, body, and soul?

_____

_____

_____

_____

_____

_____

_____

_____

What is the best way to stay focused during a mindfulness practice?

a. Noting sensations in the body
b. Refocusing attention when thoughts arise
c. Noting any physical sensations
d. All of the above

All Are Correct - Choose The Response You Feel Is Most Important To Remember

Date ___ / ___ / ___ : S   M   T   W   Th   F   S

I feel:
(please circle)

😊 because
_____
_____

😁 because
_____
_____

😋 because
_____
_____

😞 because
_____
_____

😠 because
_____
_____

Today I Am Grateful For

1. _____
2. _____
3. _____

What could help transform today into a remarkable day?

Reflective Writing

How can I cultivate a sense of curiosity and openness in my life?

_____

_____

_____

_____

_____

_____

_____

_____

What is the most important component of mindfulness practice?

a. Concentration

b. Acceptance

c. Non-judgment

d. Self-compassion

All Are Correct - Choose The Response You Feel Is Most Important To Remember

Date ___ / ___ / ___ : S M T W Th F S

I feel:
(please circle)

because _____

because _____

because _____

because _____

because _____

Today I Am Grateful For

1. _____

2. _____

3. _____

What could help transform today into a remarkable day?

Reflective Writing

What is something I can let go of or release to create more space for growth and healing?

_____

_____

_____

_____

_____

_____

_____

_____

What is the relationship between mindfulness and well-being?

a. Mindfulness can lead to a greater sense of well-being
b. Mindfulness can diminish the sense of well-being
c. Mindfulness has no impact on well-being
d. Mindfulness can increase stress and anxiety

All Are Correct - Choose The Response You Feel Is Most Important To Remember

Date ___ / ___ / ___: S   M   T   W   Th   F   S

I feel:
(please circle)

because _____   because _____   because _____   because _____   because _____

Today I Am Grateful For

1. _____
2. _____
3. _____

What could help transform today into a remarkable day?

Reflective Writing
How can I practice gratitude and appreciation in my daily life?

_____
_____
_____
_____
_____
_____
_____
_____
_____

How can mindfulness help manage stress?

a. By helping to identify and reduce stress triggers
b. By allowing for easier acceptance of difficult emotions
c. By helping to increase focus and concentration
d. All of the above

All Are Correct - Choose The Response You Feel Is Most Important To Remember

Date ___ / ___ / ___ : S M T W Th F S

I feel:
(please circle)

because _____   because _____   because _____   because _____   because _____

Today I Am Grateful For

1. _____
2. _____
3. _____

What could help transform today into a remarkable day?

Reflective Writing
What are some ways I can connect with my breath and practice mindful breathing throughout the day?

_____

_____

_____

_____

_____

_____

_____

_____

What is the difference between mindfulness and awareness?

a. Mindfulness is the practice of being aware in the present moment, while awareness is the ability to observe one's thoughts and feelings without judgment

b. Mindfulness is the practice of being aware of one's thoughts and feelings without judgment, while awareness is the ability to observe the present moment

c. Mindfulness is the practice of being aware of one's thoughts and feelings without judgment, while awareness is the ability to observe one's environment

d. Mindfulness is the practice of being aware of one's environment, while awareness is the ability to observe one's thoughts and feelings without judgment

Date ___ / ___ / ___ : S   M   T   W   Th   F   S

I feel:
(please circle)

because   because   because   because   because
_____   _____   _____   _____   _____
_____   _____   _____   _____   _____

Today I Am Grateful For

1. _____
2. _____
3. _____

What could help transform today into a remarkable day?

Reflective Writing

What is a recent mistake or setback I experienced? How can I learn and grow from it?

_____

_____

_____

_____

_____

_____

_____

54

What are some potential challenges of mindfulness practice?

a. Difficulty staying focused
b. Feeling bored or impatient
c. Feeling overwhelmed or anxious
d. All of the above

All Are Correct - Choose The Response You Feel Is Most Important
To Remember

Date ___ / ___ / ___ : S   M   T   W   Th   F   S

I feel:
(please circle)

because _____

because _____

because _____

because _____

because _____

Today I Am Grateful For

1. _____
2. _____
3. _____

What could help transform today into a remarkable day?

Reflective Writing

What are some positive affirmations or mantras I can use to empower myself?

_____

_____

_____

_____

_____

_____

_____

What is the most important thing to remember when practicing mindfulness?

a. To focus on the breath
b. To stay present in the moment
c. To be kind to yourself
d. To have no expectations

All Are Correct - Choose The Response You Feel Is Most Important To Remember

"In today's rush, we all think too much, seek too much, want too much, and forget about the joy of just being."

Eckhart Tolle

Strategies for Dealing with Stress, Anxiety, and Depression

1. Take a break. Make time for yourself to relax and do something you enjoy.
2. Exercise regularly. Exercise releases endorphins and helps reduce stress, anxiety, and depression.
3. Talk to someone. Talking to a friend, family member, or mental health professional can help you gain perspective on your situation.
4. Get enough sleep. Sleep deprivation can worsen symptoms of stress, anxiety, and depression.
5. Practice self-care. Do things you enjoy, such as taking a bath, reading a book, or going for a walk.
6. Eat a healthy diet. Eating healthy can help boost your mood and mental health.

7. Practice mindfulness. Mindfulness can help you focus on the present moment and reduce stress.

8. Set realistic goals. Setting realistic goals can help you stay motivated and reduce stress.

9. Avoid alcohol and drugs. Substance abuse can worsen symptoms of stress, anxiety, and depression.

10. Seek professional help. If symptoms of stress, anxiety, and depression persist, seek professional help from a mental health provider.

Reflective Writing

The End

As you close the pages of this mindfulness journal, remember that each word you've written is a step on your journey towards self-awareness and inner peace. Embrace the moments of clarity, the revelations, and even the uncertainties you've encountered along the way. Let this journal be a testament to your growth and a reminder that every day offers a new opportunity to be present, to observe, and to appreciate the simple wonders of life. Carry these lessons forward, and may your path be filled with mindful moments and serene reflections. Until we meet again in these pages, be gentle with yourself and stay anchored in the now.

Mindfulness isn't difficult, we just need to remember to do it.

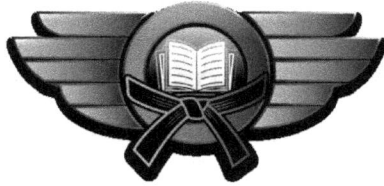

Thank You!

If you found this book helpful, I would be grateful if you would **post an honest review on Amazon** so this book can reach other supportive readers like you!

All you need to do is digitally flip to the back and leave your review. Or visit amazon.com/author/senseipauldavid click the correct book cover and click on the blue link next to the yellow stars that say, "customer reviews."

As always...
It's a great day to be alive!

**Get/Share Your FREE SSD Mental
Health Chronicles at
www.senseiselfdevelopment.care**

**Check Out The SSD Chronicles
Series CLICK HERE**

Get/Share Your FREE All-Ages Mental Health eBook Now at

www.senseiselfdevelopment.com

Or CLICK HERE

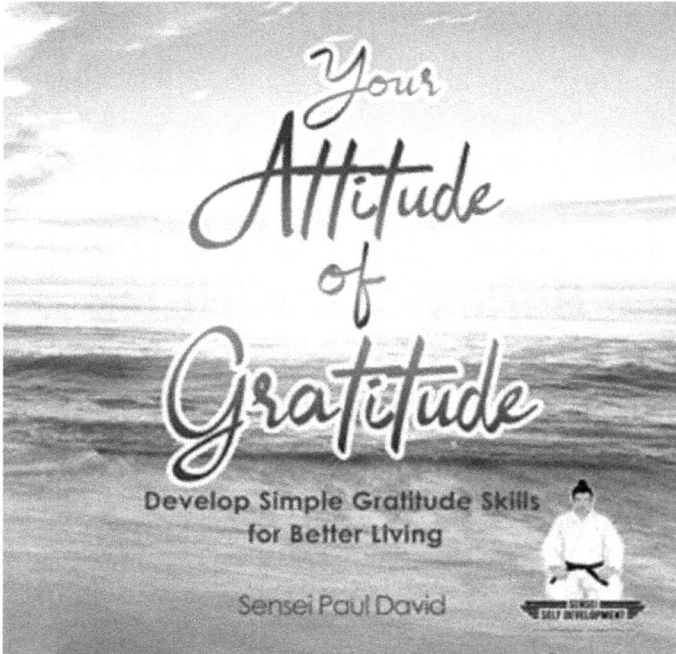

senseiselfdevelopment.com

66

Click Another Book In The SSD
BOOK SERIES:

senseipublishing.com/SSD_SERIES

CLICK HERE

SENSEI SELF DEVELOPMENT
B O O K S   S E R I E S

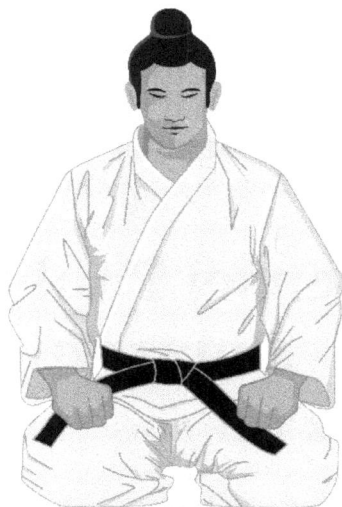

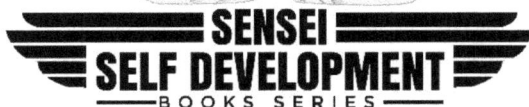

senseiselfdevelopment.senseipublishing.com

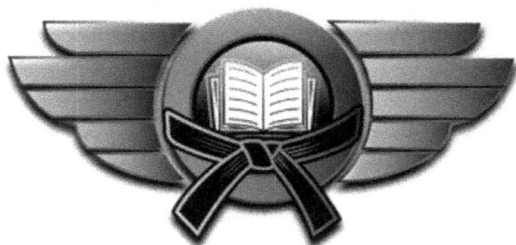

Join Our Publishing Journey!

If you would like to receive FREE BOOKS, please visit **www.senseipublishing.com**. Join our newsletter by entering your email address in the pop-up box

Follow Sensei Paul David on Amazon

CLICK THE LOGO BELOW

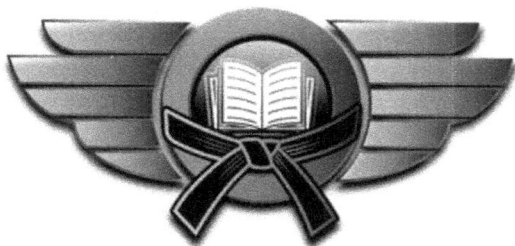

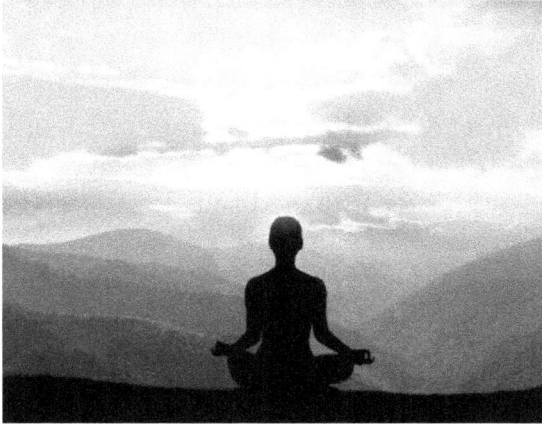

FREE BONUS!!!
Experience Over 25 FREE Engaging Guided Meditations!

Prized Skills & Practices for Adults & Kids. Help Restore Deep-Sleep, Lower Stress, Improve Posture, Navigate Uncertainty & More.

Download the Free Insight Timer App and click the link below:
http://insig.ht/sensei_paul

About Sensei Publishing

Sensei Publishing commits itself to helping people of all ages transform into better versions of themselves by providing high-quality and research-based self-development books with an emphasis on mental health and guided meditations. Sensei Publishing offers well-written e-books, audiobooks, paperbacks and online courses that simplify complicated but practical topics in line with its mission to inspire people towards positive transformation.

It's a great day to be alive!

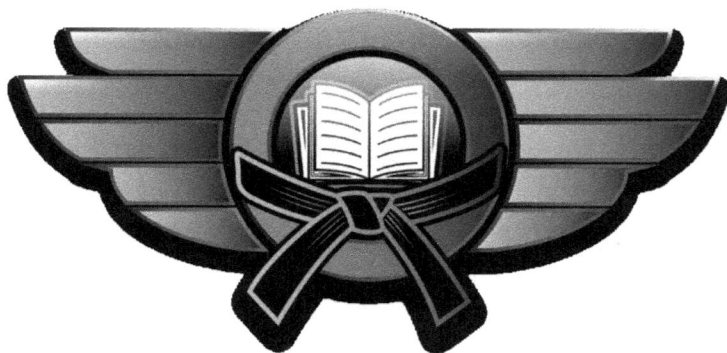

About the Author

I create simple & transformative eBooks & Guided Meditations for Adults & Children proven to help navigate uncertainty, solve niche problems & bring families closer together.

I'm a former finance project manager, private pilot, jiu-jitsu instructor, musician & former University of Toronto Fitness Trainer. I prefer a science-based approach to focus on these & other areas in my life to stay humble & hungry to evolve. I hope you enjoy my work and I'd love to hear your feedback.

- It's a great day to be alive!
Sensei Paul David

Scan & Follow/Like/Subscribe: Facebook, Instagram, YouTube: @senseipublishing

Scan using your phone/iPad camera for Social Media Visit us at www.senseipublishing.com and sign up for our newsletter to learn more about our exciting books and to experience our FREE Guided Meditations for Kids & Adults.

www.ingramcontent.com/pod-product-compliance
Lightning Source LLC
Chambersburg PA
CBHW071244020426
42333CB00015B/1625